Managing
Your Madness

A Lifestyle of Deliberate Redirection

ONE SURVIVOR'S GUIDE BY
Nanette M. Buchanan

ISBN: 978-1-0879-4466-1

This written work is not to be interpreted as a medical resource. The scenarios and examples are used to provide an explanation to the related text.

Type of Work: Non-Fiction

Creation Date: February 2021

First Edition: March 2021

Cover Design: Fideli Publishing

Published by

I Pen Books

www.NanetteMBuchanan.com

email the author at: ipendesigns@gmail.com

Foreward

If I thanked anyone for this writing, it would have to be, Corretta Doctor. After a speaking engagement, during a difficult time in my life, she simply asked did I have anything written pertaining to the topic I addressed. I hadn't given it a thought. I spoke about my mindset, the changes I made in my life, and how it had new meaning.

Setting goals, overcoming challenges, and relying on my courage had become more than the result of determination, it was the mindset I needed to get me through a difficult time. I'll discuss this further in the chapters ahead. Corretta sparked a thought, now this book. I pray it does for you, what it has done for me.

We all need to be aware of what makes us tick. When or what changes our attitude, our feelings, and how we think. How do we react physically and emotionally? Can we create the outcome we want in certain situations? This writing is not meant to be a medical resource, as I have no degree in the mental health field. However, I've worked in environments where the madness people create can affect our reactions, physically and mentally. It is our mind that interprets and hold on to our thoughts and reactions. The effects can remain with us for years.

Just as the title *Managing Your Madness* suggests, we are the owners of our madness. It, as well as our mind, is a personal possession. I suggest you keep that a forethought as you read through the pages, and in the future as well. This book is about you, just as the presentation Corretta heard was about me.

A pause in life is not meant to be the end of one's journey. What you adapt to becomes what your mind sets as its reality. Think and stay positive as your journey continues.

I hope this reading brings you peace.

Acknowledgments

To my husband, look where we are now, it has been a journey, and I thank you for your support and love. Even after retirement, planning to travel, and continuing to write…we somehow had to pause. I am blessed in knowing you and I have managed this madness. Tried and true, we have truly been blessed. As I continue to do what I love, I thank you for being a part of my inner voice. You've made what amazes me easy. I don't know if I would have ever published a book without your encouragement.

To my family and readers. Thank you for your support. I see you as the reason. Your nods of approval and words of comfort during a tough time brought tears of recognition, "I'm still here". Again, I Pen… because it's what I love to do. You read, for the same reason… what a wonderful thing.

Managing Your Madness

Your Madness

A Lifestyle of Deliberate Redirection

Table of Content

Madness: Causes & Effects

Understanding the cause and effect of one's madness has always been the question. After all, without proper diagnosis or a record of instances how is the madness confirmed? This book will not give you the answer. I won't be writing about those who are diagnosed with mental illness though I encourage all who read this work to seek medical advice if it's warranted.

The connotation of "madness" would lead one to understand that the word can be used without a medical attachment. I found three distinct definitions for madness.

1. The state of being mentally ill, especially severely.

2. Extremely foolish behavior.

3. A state of frenzied or chaotic activity.

In understanding our daily behaviors, we are not referring to the first definition. However, we all can attest to being a witness or active participant to both the second and third definitions, being foolish and a part of a frenzied, chaotic activity. We certainly can identify the behavior in others. The question is how often do we admit to our "madness" and its effect on our lives or the lives of others?

Anthony Robbins has discovered, through over forty years of experience, that there are six human needs that fundamentally affect the way we make choices. Depending on which of the basic human needs are foremost in our personality, you could be spending a lot of time consciously or subconsciously trying to meet one or two of them. And if you don't succeed, it could negatively impact your overall sense of well-being.(www.tonyrobbins.com)

These six basic human needs fulfill our emotional and psychological desires:

Certainty — The need for safety, security, comfort, order, consistency, control

Variety — The need for uncertainty, diversity, challenge, change, surprise, adventure

(The above two balance each other bringing one to a focal point)

Significance — The need for meaning, validation, feeling needed, honored, wanted, special

Love and Connection — The need for connection, communication, intimacy, and shared love with others

Growth — The need for physical, emotional, intellectual, and spiritual development

Contribution — The need to give, care, protect beyond ourselves, to serve others, and the good for all

These needs give us balance. Daily decisions, our actions and reactions, our perceptions, and interpretations, are based on these needs. It is from this aspect that I will be speaking.

Unconsciously, we seek to fulfill our needs and often it causes the madness we create. It becomes habit, affects our thoughts and mindset, it changes our actions. These needs are not determined in any order as it depends on the person, where they are in their life, and the result of any situation. Again, this "madness" is not always plotted or planned.

One's reaction as it relates to the human needs, habits, and unconscious evaluation plays a part in this "madness" …it becomes a part of our mindset. Your mindset is your way of thinking, your frame of mind. It is your life experiences, your background, culture, and education. As you grow, your thoughts, beliefs, and attitudes are formed as you process new information. Your mindset is ever changing, as will the priority of your basic needs.

The importance of each gives relevance to the decisions we make and the habits we form to protect these needs. Each requires one to have the ability to balance their living, their decisions, actions, and their "madness". After preparing myself for a lifelong change, I realized that my needs had been altered. If I couldn't prepare my mind for this permanent change, "madness" would influence my life.

STRESS

The moment situations change, you can feel it. The situation can be personal or professional, either can cause panic, fear, questions without answers, worry and distress. In the moment you are still, you don't know what to do. The reaction or actions to follow can be positive or negative, causing stress or distress.

Stress or Distress can be defined as the degree to which you feel overwhelmed or unable to cope because of pressures that are unmanageable. (www. mentalhealth.org) It's your body's response to anything that requires attention or action. How you respond makes the difference.

Eustress is the moderate or normal psychological stress interpreted as being beneficial. It's good stress, a moment of happiness. (Wikipedia) It is a healthy form of stress and gives positive feelings.

We often just say "stress" a term, that defines the negative and we give no credence to "eustress" though we face it throughout our lives as well. However, it is our reactions to the negative that is immediately connected to our subconscious, our mindset. When asked about stressors we don't often refer to celebrations, good news, or achievements. Even as we think of the good that happens it often is not a constant annoyance.

These scenarios explain both, stress/distress, and eustress. Situations don't have to be extreme, and in this case may be expected but our emotions, needs, and the result is still a part of our reaction.

Scenarios:

1. A high-school graduation can become stressful. It is a chance to celebrate an achievement but the fear of the child leaving home, the cost of college, the panic as one waits for acceptance letters, etc. are all stressors…however, it is positive, eustress stress.

2. A high school set back, the need for higher S.A.T. scores, the unknown course of the youth's future, the child who has no desire to further their education and no plans for employment, the fear of what will be next in their life are also stressors… however, this does not seem to be a temporary situation, and may cause other problems, and more distress.

One's mindset is based on the six human needs. Ask yourself are they fulfilled as described here? What human needs does either situation question? Think of yourself as the parent in this situation.

It starts with a plan. One filled with dreams, visions, and goals. You hold on to what you know, learn and experience, until...

What you're facing, the reality of the moment, that day, week, or year becomes an uncertainty- you're unsure of what's next. When there is no bounce back or balance, when you can't see beyond that point — you have no idea what it means or will mean.

In reading the second scenarios, what are the immediate thoughts that come to mind? What do they cause, and what's your first reaction?

- Panic

- Fear

- Questions without answers

- Worry

- Distress

In the moment, being the parent, you don't know how to respond. Stress has set in.

Stress can lead to unhealthy habits, thinking, and mental pressures that create serious complications that can change ones living and lifestyle. Stress can cause problems that can lead to premature death.

Stress can affect all in the home. In ages 8-17 14% of children say that adult stress doesn't really bother them. But between the ages of 15-24 in 2019 the suicide rate was 76% while from 2007-2017 in ages 10-14 the rate was 178%. The stressors varied from home to school, bullying to access to weapons and drugs, but the underlying factor is stress, pressure, fear, depression, and a list that is like adults. (www.apa.org)

Stress in adults between the ages of 34-47 averages 55% and the mature older adult joins them. After 2020, I'm sure the statistics will climb well above what they have been. Again, the uncertainty, and questions of what is and will be affect all. In 2020 all the basic human needs we discussed were altered for everyone. As one battles with stress the question becomes, what is normal?

ANXIETY

In the scenario, the student who has no plans has caused worry, nervousness, unease, a normal response when there is an uncertain outcome. As with stress, anxiety can be positive when the situation has been pre-determined, the outcome expected, and plans are in place. When there is no plan, and all becomes questionable it can lead to a negative result.

Anxiety is intense, can be excessive, and cause persistent worry and fears. Rapid breathing, sweating, an increased heart rate, can be attributed to this reaction. Even minor situations become major; Traffic jams, running late for work, an interview, moving to a new location, starting a new job, the list varies depending on an individual's mindset, reactions, and actions. Stress and Anxiety can trigger other health complications.

"MADNESS"

What makes the difference? When do we know? Most don't admit to their reactions regarding stress or having anxiety. We often feel we're "handling" things, we'll "get over it". We expect to have a response, feel a certain way, and of course, and we stand on our belief "it won't last long."

We become irritable, restless, and overwhelmed. Finding it hard to focus, we make bad decisions, are easily frustrated, and angered. We are not motivated, we lose focus, and become depressed. Guilt sets in followed by bouts of depression. It's not something that's easy to hide, yet we cover it with a smile, our determination to carry on, and the willingness to ignore the obvious. Continuing without changing our thoughts, our habits and our mind is accepting "madness".

Our habits, the norm is broken. This includes being able to maintain our health. Insomnia is usually the first indication that "something" is wrong. The inability to get adequate rest is the result of new stressors, new triggers being a part of our daily lives. Not being able to resolve matters or cause some realm of stability disrupts our subconscious. At times this will include going to bed early, realizing we are shutting down. We admit we need a moment, "a good night's rest". We reach for additives, P.M. medicine, sleep aids, maybe a drink or getting a prescription because… we just can't sleep.

Let's look again at the second scenario. As parents, we worry, we're frustrated and the senior who thinks they've got a plan is no longer listening to reasoning. The stress, aggravation, and anxiety begin to mount. Of course, this is only one facet in your life. After all you still have a family, your employment, the other children, maybe you care for an elder, I'm sure you get the idea. You're determined that this phase your child is going through will pass. After all, it did for your oldest, your best friends' daughter, and

it did for you, so you put it out of your mind…
it finds a place to nestle in your subconscious.

You've had a few headaches that seem to persist and you're still not sleeping. Conversations with your spouse no longer include the graduate, neither of you can convince the other that it will be okay. You go to the doctor only to find that your blood pressure is higher than normal, and you need to come in for a more intense examination.

This example can lead to other medical complications, heart problems, and other conditions that can be curtailed if we alleviate stressors. Again, this is not a cure, but being able to manage the intensity of our daily actions and reactions we can save ourselves from what leads to dangerous health issues.

ANGER AND FRUSTRATION

Usually when one becomes upset over minor situations after a day of chaos or overwhelming situations, we can understand their frustration. Temporary bouts of anger are also understood, and both could be a relatable response depending on the cause.

Those in our immediate circle, family, friends, and co-workers observe our actions and reactions. Often, they tell us we are stressed, needing time to relax and calm down. There are a few who can relate to our problems, they understand our reactions. The stress and our reactions are personal and relatable. At one time or another stress has taken a toll on all of us.

Anger, that annoyance or displeasure can last for a moment or be prolonged and become hostility. Fumed from actions we can't control and the frustration of being temporarily or permanently inconvenienced we seek to escape our emotions and replace them with temporary pleasures.

As this relates to our six human needs, we can find instances where when any of the needs is not fulfilled, we can become frustrated. Our balance is unstable and even if for a moment we can't control our state of mind, the "madness".

Recognizing the Behaviors and Patterns

We deny the "madness" exists when it's us, when it's others we immediately point it out to them and anyone who will discuss it or listen. Why? Human nature? No one wants to be labeled as being unable to handle their problems. Large or small, we want to say we managed the situation. The truth is not all situations are manageable. There will be times when the situation is not for us to control. "The Serenity Prayer" comes to mind for me whenever I find myself facing a situation that I can't step away from nor am I able to handle at that time.

I've realized not ever situation has an immediate solution. Circumstances may warrant time, or others to be involved. One may find they just don't have the means to handle the problem at hand. Often, we accept the outcome, though it may be only for that moment, and continue without a resolution.

We all have heard or said: *"It's going to be one of those days."*

At that point, the person speaking has put the thought of a "bad" day in their subconscious. It becomes the excuse, the reason for any problem that may happen as the day goes on... and it's just 8:00 in the morning. How could they know how the day will turn out because they got caught in traffic, spilled their coffee, or the office phone rang more than twice before they sat down. The message sent is from their innate defense. The attitude changes prepared for the next problem. They will challenge the next problem they're confronted with no matter how big or small it may be. By the end of the day, they're exhausted because they've been hyped throughout the day prepared to defend whatever confronts them.

They are reassuring their basic human need. Certainty, significance, growth… at least three of the needs we've discussed fall into the reasoning for the change of attitude. Although the morning traffic triggered this attitude there's underlying stress, frustration and maybe anger that is crying out. The "madness" is exposing itself, yet they can't see it.

There are many who need that moment in the morning to, what I call, armor up. The cup of coffee, the early exercise routine, prayer, and yoga, we'll discuss a few of these later. These are people who have learned to manage or try to manage their madness. Without the morning habits, they too have the morning grouch attitude.

I am a functional morning person, but I will admit my personality doesn't kick in until mid-morning, 10 a.m. Today, I talk about my mindset but this habit, recognizing my morning personality started in high school. Once recognized, I stopped blaming the happenings during the day on a "bad" morning, least of all one I was responsible for creating. I would say that this was my first step toward aligning myself with positive thinking.

Recognizing the behaviors and patterns of the madness we harbor within is as difficult as recognizing it in those we care for. Loving or having admiration for another keeps us from admitting their bad behaviors or the habits that are rooted in their stressors. We may make mild references to what we assume is their problem. "You drink too much", "You don't get enough rest", but that's the result of an embedded problem.

Remember there is that "other" definition for madness. There may be situations where we and/or those we love will need a professional, therapy, and treatment to help us manage our "madness". We may need a professional to peel back the layers and identify the stressor that has caused the results that are slowly damaging us.

When it is unmanageable the effect can lead to serious health issues that can affect all involved.

MALADAPTIVE/IRRATIONAL THINKING

Our behavior pattern is based on how we act as an individual as well as how we adapt when in a group. As humans, we adapt accordingly. To fit in, survive, overcome, thrive, to meet those six basic human needs, we adapt. Psychology explores behavior patterns. This vast information relates to the relationship between our behavior and our mindset. Our habits and routines become who we are as well as the patterns that define us to others.

Maladaptive Thinking refers to a belief that is false and rationally unsupported. It is easy to believe that after having a bout with stress, depression, and insomnia, one may have convinced themselves that "bad things" are always going to be a part of their life. One may feel detached from family, friends, co-workers, and people. They disconnect themselves from positive thinking or the thought of being worth positive outcomes.

Irrational Thinking refers to giving a conclusion, action, or opinion without a use of reason. This type of thinking causes one to easily get annoyed or nervous. Putting the blame on others, refusing to follow rules, arguing, and having difficulty handling frustration. Fear is baseline for this type of thinking and being challenged causes the flight or fright mentality.

Recognizing what causes fear, panic, anger, and frustration is a plus. I can't over emphasize that therapy and treatment should be sought when a pattern of these behaviors has become one's norm. Stress and anxiety mounted with these patterns can cause unmanageable situations when overlooked and ignored.

These triggers and the patterns they form become obvious. We no longer need someone to say, "I'm upset", "It's been a bad day", etc. We see it in their expression, it's displayed in their actions, we recognize the signs of their "good times" and "bad times". Once negative behaviors are displayed many ignore a need to alert the person that they need help. No one wants the confrontation, arguments, or aggressive responses. The support and concern rejected; the advice ignored. People often describe them as disgruntle, uncooperative, hard to work with… the list goes on.

MALADAPTIVE/IRRATIONAL THINKING PATTERNS

- **All or nothing** — Perfect or not at all attitude

- **Mental filter** — See failures, ignore success, focus on one thing more than others

- **Over analyzing** — Creating a pattern based on one single event (if it happened before, it will happen again)

- **Assumptions** — believing without proof or evidence

Negative thoughts promote negative actions and reactions. When one's thinking pattern has become diminished with stress, doubt, and depression, their mental pattern is maladaptive.

The point I am making here is adapting a positive mindset must become a daily habit. We must redirect our way of thinking by feeding our subconscious and conscious mind positive rational thoughts. Our conscious mind feeds from our subconscious and when we create positive habits and reflections, we change our mindset, our "madness" to a lifestyle we can control.

THE MIND — CONSCIOUS/SUBCONSCIOUS

Certain regions of the brain become hyperactive during a panic attack. Chronic stress can cause anxiety and cause damage to the brain. It can lead to depression and a risk for other problems even dementia and other psychiatric disorders. (www.sciencedaily.com)

There may be many things in life that cause panic and fear. Many we adapt to; we know how to react or calm ourselves when it occurs.

- Emotional reaction
- Remaining calm
- Just stand

Through a mental process we often can break down a situation before it becomes overwhelming.

Our subconscious doesn't work separately. It follows the thoughts of the conscious mind. It takes six weeks to reprogram the thoughts held in your subconscious. Bad habits can take up to a year or longer. Your subconscious mind must be changed from negative to positive before the conscious mind will react accordingly.

The subconscious is fed by your habits. Your conscious awareness of your decisions, actions, and emotions and behavior depends on 95% of what is programmed in your subconscious.

How did you react to the problem or situation before? What emotional connection do you have to the problem? Your reaction will determine if your emotions will be reset or recognized to remain the same.

With positive thoughts, and uplifting ideas, your subconscious will begin to implement a positive pattern for your conscious mind to follow.

- Change — It is the response needed to move on

- Relationships — both distant and close

- Work

- Home Life

"What could possibly change the mess I'm facing?" Some would respond to their own question "That's madness…it's just easier to settle and adapt to the madness." Their mind is set, they've accepted… what they've already accepted and identified as "madness" …mindset madness.

Those of us who see them, interact with them daily, have our own perception of their struggle… "Oh, they're crazy!" With just a thought we've adapted to their behavior, accepted they won't change. This is the slippery slope.

MINDSET DISPARITIES

Our decisions and actions are based on what we think because of our social status, culture, race, and belief system. Could these differences cause irrational comparisons, false interpretations, and unjust disparities? Could the six basic human needs be different because of these disparities?

The mindset, becomes hardened, protective of those needs and seeking to be equal on some level. "Madness" comes with constant comparisons, living up to expected standards, the persistent expectations of others. We've discussed that path to "madness".

How does one guard and protect themselves, their basic human needs when the "madness" is prevalent on so many levels?

- Ancestral History

- Racial/Social Differences

- Poverty/Economical

- Education Levels/Labels

- Therapy Feats/Defeats/Phobias

- Family Setbacks/History

- Social Delusion/Inclusion

- Poor Self-Image

- Mental Lock-Up/Mental breakdown

As a minority, I often joke about my "disparities". As real as they are my mindset won't allow me to settle for what others believe I am or will do based on their interpretations. Although these disparities are as real for me as they are for others. I find myself above the norm.

My gender, my age, marital status, children? No great differences there, let's continue. My ethnicity, income, my education level... now we're beginning to separate me from others. My family history, medical history, and of course the "have you ever"?

Let me explain, many applications, request for documents, or screenings lead to the disparities that cause people of color, those of foreign decent, to stress.

Once we fill out applications, visit a doctor, wait for approval, compete for a score, are called a minority, we recognize the process, and understand the fate. Labels may put us ahead when grants, money and politics are involved, but there are labels that we wear a lifetime that set us back.

Generational disparities, just like health conditions don't get diagnosed. They are accepted barriers. Habits, addictions, the unwillingness to do more, we live with what many believe is the norm. The expectations in the inner cities are not the same as they are in the rural areas. Our fight, the fight of those identified by the labels is with the system and the stress of everyday norms.

"You're a strong black woman". This statement is not always meant as a compliment, it's often an expectation. One that often means we don't need the support or help from anyone, especially our men. We as the woman who has stood alone and succeeded, will survive. This preconceived notion has separated our families, caused the breakdown in our ability to be a strong unit for our children, and left us without the basic lifestyle others have at birth. Evidence that we are not expected to be much more than our predecessors, even after all the history, years gone by, there are many who believe and live daily without expectations of living a life of peace and comfort...without the "madness".

The interpretation of who we are, and the expectations of others based on disparities causes reactions and actions. Labels, denials, racial tension, and the need for basic medical intervention often causes fear, panic, and denial. "When you know better…" The problem is most don't know.

Just the thought of it all questions our world, how we live, and how we continue to survive. The pressures bring on the problems that can mount from subtle to major. The outcome…the "madness".

Madness Without Support

When the "madness" within becomes over-powering the need to escape becomes imminent. Friends and family are usually the first to observe there is a problem. They may offer support, advice alternatives, or in many cases fill in the missing role. Family members, outside of the home, become parents, counselors, doctors, they compensate for what's missing. If the individual who is overwhelmed with stress, anxiety and all that follows won't admit their problems, the "madness" can escalate.

Those closest to the individual are affected daily. Their coping methods are laced with stress as well. As they watch the "madness" spiral they must be aware of how to handle their reaction and actions. The sooner they recognize the problems and make appropriate changes the better for all.

We've described the behaviors of many as being mad without recognizing without change we all would be described as "mad."

- Relationship and family issues

- Loss of Job/Financial Setbacks

- Depression

- Addictions

- Binging Habits

- Fear/Avoidance

- Guilt

- Suicide/Domestic Violence

- PTSD

- Health Concerns

Each of these situations, including mindset disparities can and has promoted generational madness. These issues become the normal, a way of life, a part of community culture. Continuing to live this way should not be accepted as the norm and it can be avoided.

Our actions and how we react is controlled by our minds. We control or allow others to control our thoughts…positive or negative. Our acceptance of either becomes what leads us on.

Scenarios:

1. The community shelter has opened its doors to anyone who finds themselves without shelter or food. Keeping those who are within their walls safe is a priority. The funding is based solely donations and community outreach programs. Liz and her two children have been at the shelter for two weeks. Each day she gets dressed from the clothes she's packed in her car, her children are off to school, and she begins her search for a job. Although she has been a victim of Domestic Vio-

lence, had her bout with guilt, depression, anger, and frustration, she seeks to achieve.

2. Elaine lives at the shelter. She is determined that it is her fate, the result of drugs, a bad marriage, and abandoning her children. She believes she will never do better. She doesn't talk much to those living in the center, but Elaine sparks her attention. Elaine meets Liz each day as she returns from her job searches with a discouraging word or comment and a promise to share her stories. Elaine spends her days drinking. She makes money here and there working the food banks. She convinces Liz it's a day's pay and she shouldn't be so picky. After weeks of failed job searches, Liz agrees to go with Elaine to the food banks. While working with Elaine, Liz finds they have more in common than not.

After months of working together Liz finds work and brings an application to Elaine.

The relationship between the ladies changes the scope of support. Neither has reason to criticize the other, but they do for the first few weeks of their meeting. However, after talking, learning from the other's experience they find they can help each other, give advice and support. Their mindset changed. Liz was seeking to escape while Elaine was content. The improvement of their attitudes worked in favor for the two of them. Imagine the conversations, the changes they both made to redirect their lives. What human needs were they fulfilling living in the shelter? What human needs did they fulfill by working at the food bank? What influence did they have on each other?

Today, oppression looms over the heads of many. The anticipated help from many authorities has shattered families, removed fathers from homes and created everlasting fears. The assistance and help in many communities are at risk as resources become scarce. The result of what most simply label as crisis is a way of life for those who have adapted to "doing without".

Our acceptance influences our actions. Although years have passed since the "Depression", many live the era generation after generation. Unlike Liz and Elaine, we no longer share our personal business with the neighbor, we no longer share our conditions or complain to others. In humor and jest we mock those who are fighting the results. We belittle those who attempt to achieve and fail. We have become cold to those who stay in situations we've overcome or moved away from.

Once we've conquered a problem, tackled a situation we seem to believe we're above others. This behavior complicates and compounds the negative results one experiences. Family matters can be torn and long lasting, depression, addictions and binging habits increase. This cycle repeats and becomes permanent and as the sub-conscious prepares us for the next, our reaction is the same. Our health is not the better for it. Therapy is recommended for anyone suffering from any mental disorder, suicide ideation, long lasting depression and/or guilt, domestic violence, and PTSD.

Post-Traumatic Stress Disorder is thought to be a major problem for those serving in the military. This disorder affects anyone who has suffered from a severe traumatic encounter. Either as a witness or participant the subconscious has processed the situation and protected those involved the best it can. However, flashbacks nightmares, severe anxiety and uncontrollable thoughts recur. When one cannot control the situation, change the circumstance, they can't find peace. It creates mental chaos, and the mindset is disrupted, and negative actions are often the result.

Reveal & Heal

REVEAL

Identifying and understanding there is a problem, while determining the cause, and resolution is easier said than done. Stating what it is, saying it to yourself awakens the mind to find a solution. Being silent won't provoke action; speaking with others may cause vulnerability. However, admitting the need for support or advice is a positive step in overcoming the problems that surface from baseline stressors.

Tell the truth, the whole truth, to yourself. Admitting your full participation in the situation is important and must be handled with care. Revealing your part in the matter is not the same as having a "pity" party or sitting in a moment of depression. Often, we don't realize our contribution to our own stress. It comes disguised as caring, being helpful, getting the job done. I'm sure you can relate to many of the excuses we often use without facing the reality.

If you are stressing about a task that you feel is not your job, question how you were assigned the task, you may have to face facts. Often, we volunteer our services or help without recognizing we put ourselves in an unwanted situation. If the stress has been caused by another's actions that involve us, we must confront them regarding the situation. Ask the appropriate questions and only those that involve your participation.

Scenario:

1. Kari works as an assistant to the Sales Representatives desk on her job. While each of the other assistants is assigned three to four representatives, Kari has been doing the work of two and sometimes three assistants. You see Kari has a scheduled time to complete each of her

tasks during the day. There have been times while Kari is making copies for her Sales desks, another assistant will want to cut between her job just to get a "copy" or "two". The other assistants watch and wait for Kari to go to the copy machine and are now dropping off their copies at her desk to be done as well.

Kari didn't notice until Bill, a Sales Representative that Kari didn't work for, asked where were his copies? He expressed that he was getting them later and later and could she manage to copy his in the morning instead of waiting until the end of the day. Kari had taken on the job of preparing the copies and was expected by not just Bill but others to perform the task.

Kari thought a simple email would clear up the matter among herself and the other assistants. No one answered the email and the following week, Bill and two other Sales Representatives met her at the copy machine to ask why their copies were not stapled and collated as requested. They informed her that the job was better performed before she was assigned to handle it.

Kari took the office stress home with her in the car each day. It clouded her decisions when she arrived each morning. No matter how she rearranged her workload her basket on her desk was now the drop-off for copies, with notes indicating what was to be done.

After spending her lunch hour a few days to clear up the job, her Sales Representative noticed she hadn't taken a break. When he called her in the office, and she explained how she got overwhelmed he called for an office meeting. Kari presented a schedule that would fit for all the assistants to use the copier, and another representative suggested the purchase of another copier.

Kari needed to speak up. She had begun to dread coming in the office. She was uncomfortable with the Sales Teams, and her co-workers seemed pleased with her misery.

During my employment, in all positions, I've often found my advancement was based on being willing to work above and beyond my title. It also included learning positions that didn't necessarily define the work I did daily or was expected to do. This caused others to spread rumors and gossip about my intent. They never asked questions or wanted to be a part of the training or assist with the workload. This would make some days difficult. Working with disgruntle co-workers or employees who were intent on stopping me from "doing so much".

My reaction, I'll admit, made me hesitant when I was confronted with the realities and their attitudes toward me. I wanted to be a part of the team, I often wasn't included in conversations or the laughs within the office or during assignments. However, my movement through the departments, accepting new challenges and positions, painted new pictures for me. My mindset changed. I found there were others who noted my ability to rise above the normal expectations. It benefitted me as well as the supervisors. I was offered opportunities that weren't extended to others.

I didn't openly admit that their subliminal messages, actions, and reactions caused stress. As truthful as I was with myself and my family, I still felt detached. Often, I had to remind myself that I would be better, and not bitter. It wasn't easy but with the support of family, and those I worked for, I learned that you can only control your actions. It was about what I wanted in my career, and what I accepted would affect my reactions. I leaned on the advice given, said the serenity prayer, and managed my "madness."

Talking about your matters, that which you hold close to you, can be difficult. No one wants to admit personal problems. Their health, marriage, family, and the pitfalls are not a conversation we can trust everyone to hold and be silent about. Minorities, especially African Americans, have a phobia when it comes to therapy.

However, today, everyone is willing to talk with a "Life Coach", aka a business or personal therapist. I find it quite interesting. All the problems we find in business are not based on the lack of finance, employees, or being overwhelmed. Building a business has its own stressors.

Our problems at home find a way to ride to work with us. Our problems at work, well they come back home at the end of the day. Simply, if we could stuff the "madness" in a jar I'm sure not many of us would open that jar and retrieve it. Revealing whatever it is… changes things.

The discussion gives permission to what we've been keeping secret. Surprise! Most people know the problem and have been waiting for someone to say what it is aloud. Make a choice… a comfortable choice. If we tell the truth, we can make the comfortable choice. The choice, feels good when we say it aloud, "I can't do this anymore!"

That outcry, yell, scream is often done in our mind, the subconscious. It is the reaction that needs to be guided. "What's next?" A drink, a drug, binging habits; insomnia, depression, headaches. The cycle begins over and over ending with the same questions until we reveal there is a serious problem. Stating what it is to our support, telling them we can't handle this alone, sharing and listening to another is the first step to healing.

Release the fears. Let go of the struggle. There are times when we struggle, we question is it better to ignore how we feel to avoid problems with others. We become silent in our feelings, sighing deeply as we find an excuse to hide behind. I've mentioned what the stress, without releasing the fears, or managing the madness, can become.

There's no bandage that covers a wound that hasn't been tended to. The wound must be thoroughly cleaned, if necessary prepped and stitched so it can heal. The wounds created the hurt that has been carried for years, the pain that has settled in our subconscious needs more. It starts with our mind recognizing the hurt, the struggle, and how we've been covering our wounds.

Our fear to let go is often entangled with our fear of change. We may have to look for other employment, leave a home, a marriage, or a friendship. We may have to find our voice, speak up, or set new rules and conditions.

We may have to be more discipline regarding our habits, restrictions, and be firm in our rejections. We may have to seek support, professional help, but we must commit ourselves to change.

HEAL

Healing is never short term. It's an ongoing process, a change, and time does not manage progress. Managing your "madness" starts with change. Our pain, baseline stressors are deeply rooted in our subconscious. They are joined with the habits and alternatives we've conformed to change often in a temporary moment of needed relief. The peace and comfort that healing brings is woven in our determination to heal.

Revealing our problems, facing the challenges and self-talk are starting points. The voice must be strong when speaking a "new" language. We can no longer be okay with being passive. Making better choices for ourselves daily starts with a healthy thought process.

Creating new habits, avoiding stressors, stepping out of our comfort zone will become a part of the daily routine if we learn and apply limits. The willingness to detach ourselves from old habits without reattaching to old norms, is a challenge. The habits that we don't even recognize is again the subconscious feeding the conscious mind.

The people we no longer speak to and places we no longer go; we avoid them because of past encounters, the memories that caused issues and problems. We learn avoidance because of the past mistakes, stressors. We detach, praying not to reattach, there is a feeling of freedom. We need to hone the ability to breathe it, speak it, and go through it without shame.

At times it's the conversations, the willingness to share, the desire to let others know that you have found the pain and a cure. Often, we celebrate before we fully recover, before we've walked away without looking back before we've changed.

SETBACKS

Expect setbacks, the healing is real once you pass the temptation to revert to old habits. Accepting others as they are includes accepting their habits, however, understand if they infringe on your healing their actions should not be accepted. Growth and healing are entwined in the saying *"People come into your life for a reason, a season or a lifetime." When you figure out which one it is, you will know what to do for each person.* (www.selinamankarisson.com)

The problem is we often hold on well past the season. When it begins to be uncomfortable, we either settle in and ignore the quirks of stress or we move on. We often find the need to "find ourselves" and leave the situations longing for relief only after the irritation has set in. Our habits of acceptance also wear on the conscious mind, knowing the relationship may be unhealthy mentally, physically, and spiritually.

Change is the breakthrough. The aggravation mounts and the irritation will push until you are no longer comfortable with what has become your tolerable new norms. Your job, your home, your family, your friends, can encourage you to push through it, but until you're uncomfortable, unhealthy, tired, and frustrated, change won't be real. The irritation touches deep, it goes against your beliefs, your understandings and you can't recognize the reason you've accepted the annoyance this long.

Take the time to reflect, the stressors, how did it start? You will tell yourself it doesn't matter; the irritation is telling you it must stop. Your breakthrough, the small changes in your habits has shown you possibilities. You have peeped into what could be a new reality. You've lost a few pounds, you're sleeping better, you don't have the headaches daily, you and your family are communicating, it's possible you can move on. You've reduced your some of the stress. Irritation has raised your awareness; you can now see the next step in your life. The subconscious is holding on to your fears.

We all back away. It's that voice, it reminds us of our past mistakes, it tells us what we know is safer than any of the unknown. We can control the stressors that are our norms, how will we control the unknown? Can we hide the fears that cause us to binge, lose sleep, snap at our family, can we? Are we stressing as we fight the battles of our past? Irritation…

Agitation brings on anxiety, this too is a natural part of healing. We question the fears, we question our actions, we are working against what feels better, we are no longer giving in to the norms. Breathe through it, speak through it, hold on to nothing, there is no shame in pushing through it and controlling the "madness". Release and let go.

We all have similar situations, similar problems. We don't always come through it or resolve them in the same manner. There is no quick fix or healing when "madness" has taken control of your daily life. Changing, becoming positive can and will include support. Family, friends, professionals, can give us the support that will thwart a setback.

As careful as we are about guarding our personal feelings, we must be willing to tell the truth to our support. Revealing our situations to the right person(s) or health care provider is a sensitive matter. Our "madness" creates these fears which are real and can't be ignored. Support and advice though it may be needed, is not always welcomed, or coming from the best source.

There is also that advice that we don't want to hear. Most of our healing sits on us listening to those who have forewarned us about our "madness". "You need to change...", "Why haven't you...", "How long before you...". Even from the doctor, "You have to take your medication, lose weight, get rest, change your habits."

We've heard it all before. What makes it so difficult to follow through? Setbacks, habits, fears, but there are solutions. All is not lost when we focus on deliberate changes and alternatives.

Deliberate Changes

Whenever there is change it causes a ripple effect. A simple change in one's driving route, to and from work; not stopping at the bar on the way home; scheduling family time; listen to your inner thoughts and what others have to say intently. Minor changes can begin to feel good.

Breathe through it. What doesn't make a difference often doesn't matter. We spend a lot of time being that difference for others and forgetting what would make a difference for us. We offer advice, give support, and we even step in, act, and solve major problems…for others. We must convince ourselves that change is not to be feared. It's the same fears that we work through with those we support and advise.

What changes do we expect others to make for us when we can't make those changes for ourselves?

Remember those basic needs we spoke about:

- Certainty

- Variety

- Significance

- Love and Connection

- Growth

- Contribution

Each of these, as you begin to understand the necessary changes, must be met to give you balance in your life. We're not secure without fulfilling our needs. I mention this to remind you that the stressors we allow in our daily lives question that balance. To maintain these basic skills, we fall victim to our habits good or bad.

I'm a planner. Knowing my schedule, keeps me balanced. Just like everyone, there are days when I don't have anything planned or emergencies come up. On most days, I plan the days, times, and locations. It is important for me. I avoid the stress of rushing, being late, or missing appointments or events. This habit was formed well before I began my first job. It started in school. Being late for class, practice, or turning in assignments were reported to my parents. It had its repercussions and it affected others. Late class brought one after school detention; late for practice to any sport would afford me extra laps, exercise, or not being able to be in the next game or competition; turning in assignments late had an effect on my grades. A warning was given for excused lateness, but it was frowned upon.

The punishment, though I rarely fell victim to any, kept me on schedule. Stressed? That's questionable, but as an adult I didn't want to know the punishment. Would I be rushing to work in traffic? Would I have a problem on the job? Would I be late picking up my children? Would I be late filing important paperwork? The list of possibilities seems endless. To avoid it all, I'm rarely late and if so, there's a valid reason.

Anxiety brings on headaches, a problem I've had since childhood. I never thought of my migraines as a part of anxiety. However, excitement or surprise, sudden changes, good or bad news, I may have an episode. I've learned to recognize it, try to remain calm and worry less. I had to accept and try to control this untamed emotion. It's been years and I still have moments filled with anxiety.

Deliberate changes are necessary to avoid the outcomes we are sure will happen. I don't rush, often if I have to rush, I'll cancel to avoid the stress and anxiety. Being sick because of the rush isn't worth it for me. I make the necessary changes to avoid the outcome and my internal conflict.

There's plenty of sayings about listening to others, arguing your point, or avoiding known conflict. I used these sayings daily though they didn't make sense in my youth… "with age come wisdom."

A few of my favorites deal with communication. Stress is often rooted in conversations. People want to get their point across and will defend themselves as they attempt to communicate.

- *"It's not a conversation if all parties are speaking."*

- *"You can't understand if you won't listen."*

- *"No one can argue by themselves."*

Remembering these, allow me to avoid most arguments and confrontations. I've found that the two basic needs *"certainty and love and connection"* live within our communication. How we express ourselves, argue a point, or just want to be heard depends on both needs. Stress becomes a factor when we can't obtain what we need at the conclusion of the communication. Being understood matters and it depends on the type of relationship we have with the person we're communicating with.

We may talk to the mailman about not receiving our mail or complain to the Postmaster. It doesn't compare to speaking with your spouse or loved one about not mailing an important letter on time.

Both can be minor stressors; both can be resolved. Stacked on other stressors one may need alternatives.

Alternatives

Our health matters. We carry our "madness", the habits of the mind, with us hoping for change. We pray for things to get better daily. We believe the problem isn't us. I must agree, for the most part, its not. We are, however, are the culprits in mismanaging our behavior, thoughts, and mindset. Prayers are answered but remember, *"God helps those who... help themselves."*

We want to feel better, do better, be better as we live, love, and share our lives with others. Our "madness" has developed over the years and its not easy to change the subconscious. We try to eat healthy, get to bed early, keep our doctor appointments, exercise...and the list can be never-ending. However, none will become habit without deliberate changes to our mindset.

A positive mind, positive thoughts take being willing to admit that our way of living may not benefit us mentally or physically. None of the following suggestions are easy. There may be other techniques, exercises, or routines that can be added to those listed here. Remember, not everything fits everyone. You may want to get a personal trainer, coach, therapist, or any other professional advice.

PRAYERS, MEDITATION, YOGA

Starting the day with meditation or prayer is a habit I adapted years ago. It doesn't have to be connected to any particular religious belief. Becoming aware that there is a higher authority, making a spiritual connection, talking to that inner voice or spirit can start your morning with a jolt of awareness. Moments of meditation, breathing exercises, stretching, and reflecting can prepare you mentally for the day and bring a resolve to the days prior. Yoga is practiced for health and relaxation. Calming the mind, body, and soul, it helps achieve a peaceful body and mind while managing stress. A morning routine can start the day by rejuvenating your system.

HEALTHY EATING HABITS — REGULAR DOCTOR APPOINTMENTS

An 8 oz. glass of water first thing in the morning immediately helps rehydrate the body. Having a balanced diet — fruits, vegetables, dairy, grains, and protein protects the body against certain types of diseases. As we get older there may be a need to change our eating habits and visit our doctors regularly. Monitoring our weight, sleep, and medication needs, helps to keep us balanced.

Our mental health is just as important. Eight hours of sleep, exercise, deep breathing exercise and a healthy breakfast keeps the brain healthy. Minimizing stress daily, volunteering and helping others, acts of kindness, having a pet or hobby can bring comfort to daily routines. Keep in mind that some mental conditions are serious and should be diagnosed by a certified physician.

EXERCISE

Many join a gym, schedule a time during the day, or meet up with friends to exercise as a group. It's an individual's choice. There are a range of exercises for all ages and conditions. Walking, stretching and even dancing can help one with their weight loss, muscle toning, sleep, and reducing stress.

Exercising to relieve stress is quite popular. Often people substitute time in the gym, a walk or jog with going to the bar for the drink, arguing with the family or spouse, or taking drugs. Clearing the mind while exercising the body often releases the frustration, anger or the "madness" that pushes the aggravation packed in a day.

It may seem hard to begin the regiment of exercising on a schedule. The saying, *"No pain, no gain"* is real. I can confess, I've made more excuses about when to start than I can count. It's a habit I need to adapt for all the reasons explained here. The pain moves on as the body adapts to each exercise. As the mind adjusts to the change, exercise gets easier. We can walk a longer distance, change the weights, and add new exercises. As we meet our goals with an exercise schedule, our stress, health, and attitude become manageable. The change needed is in the subconscious mind. That nudge, twinge or positive thought, the eustress instead of distress that will remind you it's time to release tension. A release of the day's madness, with each exercise can make you feel better about yourself knowing you have achieved a goal that you set…for you.

Scheduling me time also helps the mental and emotional state of mind. Often, we work for the good of all. Our family, friends even co-workers benefit from us being there. Taking time for ourselves is slim to none. There are those who claim it's a loving sacrifice. But don't we love ourselves enough to set aside time to do absolutely nothing or schedule a day of relaxation?

A spa day, a day on the golf course, reading a book, the barber shop or salon, an afternoon massage - We all know where to go and what to do. We make excuses due to self-imposed constraint of time or a feeling of guilt. We don't have to rush, nothing is stopping us from relaxing our minds, body, and souls…if only once a week. Vacationing once a year is fine, but for most it includes the family. The children, the spouse, friends, and when we arrive home, we need a vacation day after the vacation. We need a day where there are no repercussions if we miss a scheduled time. Me time is just for us and what we want to do. It shouldn't cause more stress. Our mind should be filled the desires on our bucket list.

Inspiration

Inspiration moves mountains. You can and will manage your madness. You will find that the peace it brings makes you aware of the madness that surrounds you daily. Unfortunately, each person must control their madness with the same determination you've made. There will always be those who doubt, or argue, they're not stressed, burned out, or "mad". Each of us has to come to realize our need for relief, the need to admit there is an irritation. Remember it takes time, truth, and patience.

However, we can inspire others, we can be the support they need. We can show them the alternatives, offer our support, share with them our experience. Letting others know you've walked the same path, not in their shoes, but in the same direction. We can tell them when we became aware of our subconscious thoughts and how they affect the willingness to change. Explaining our pains, irritants, aggravation and how to let go is important. Remembering your setbacks, expectations and reflections can help another along the way.

No one can expect you to be an authority, but *"Experience is the best teacher"*. Everyone thinks it only happens to them until they open-up to others. If someone feels comfortable enough to discuss their situation, what they don't quite understand, or how to change their direction to you, take it as a compliment. Remember what I said about trusting others. How you evaluate your supporters is how you will be evaluated. Inspire, don't prescribe. Suggesting medical attention is better than prescribing medication. You don't want to be at fault or responsible for a wrong diagnosis. If you suspect there's a problem, encourage them to seek professional help.

You know your problems; you've identified the causes. Even deep-rooted problems must be handled properly. Finding a source of inspiration can help you and those who are connected to you. Today, there's many inspirational books written by religious leaders, social groups, television shows, webinars, and conferences headed by groups and speakers. Just like health clubs, and fitness groups it's beneficial to keep yourself connected to what keeps you uplifted. Reading books, journaling, joining groups and organizations that encourage positive living and inspiration can help one maintain a positive mindset and lifestyle.

"Managing Your Madness" must become a deliberate redirection. Our journey is not based on a timeline we've created. We can't live our best life filled with stress, anxiety, frustration, and anger. Fearing change delays happiness and peace…peace of mind.

Fearing possibilities, the unknown, often can't be avoided. Death, family issues, finances, can't be predetermined. The madness that follows can be short lived if our reaction is to face it for what it is. The 2020 COVID pandemic showed us that often the "madness" becomes a contagion. The fears of others spread when faced with a crisis all based on our basic needs.

We can all attest that the sudden disruption in our lives shocks our norms. Business, educational institutions, politics and the constituents, medical and law enforcement personnel, nursing homes, travel and employment has all been affected. Not being able to meet basic needs has brought on a "different kind" of madness.

The shock that is associated with fears we can't handle can leave us paralyzed. The pandemic, death in the family, a medical diagnosis, these added to other stressors can cause mental distress. Having a positive mindset or, managing our madness may not be enough… we all need support. Someone to talk to, the alternatives, inspiration, personal strengths to pull us through, adapting to new norms. Determination, courage, love, and the awareness that we can't control everything makes a difference.

While working in the New Jersey Department of Corrections I learned to check policies, contractual agreements, and any political changes that would affect my benefits. I started my exit research and plans ten years prior to my twenty-fifth year. My husband and I did the same with personal plans, sale of our home, moving to another state, making the necessary personal and medical changes.

I received a call from my physician who called to inform me that I needed to come into his office. The conversation was brief and disheartening. I was diagnosed with cancer. Fear, anxiety, and the questions, "How?", "Why?", "When?", "What now?" followed. Reflecting on those days that followed, the diagnosis and the treatment a blur. Sleepless nights, I didn't want to talk with anyone afraid that they would tell horrid stories that I would relate to or fantasize about not having an alternative or cure. The support groups were depressing, and no family member could or speak to my imagined fate.

I hadn't changed any plans. I relocated to another state, changed medical professionals, went to scheduled events and continued to write and publish my work. I decided my condition wouldn't change my attitude. I kept the bad feelings, my questions, discussions with my husband to a minimum. I didn't want anyone to feel the way I did. Six weeks, every day… fifteen minutes of radiation and the thirty-minute drive there and back. The wait before they'd call me in totaled forty-five minutes of fear.

I walked in after my fourth week mentally drained. The receptionist signed me in, smiled and said I didn't look the way I normally did. I replied, "I didn't retire to this. Cancer was not a part of my plan." She asked did I need a social worker. I didn't catch on when she said it but reflecting later, I understood her concern. Maybe I needed that professional support, maybe I didn't want to continue my treatments, maybe my agitated response revealed my prolonged fears. She didn't know but she understood.

I explained I had after-retirement plans and cancer, well I was called in for treatment. We never finished that conversation. Paying attention to my medical needs, following a retirement plan, I was able to prevent a serious bout' with cancer. I had to have surgery to remove the cancer. Today, I am a survivor.

I will forever attest that without a deliberate redirection of my "madness", I may have slipped into severe depression. I have my days, it's not always easy, I've adjusted to new norms. I'm certain a positive mind, changing habits and being aware of my fears has brought me through a trying time in my life.

Managing my madness kept me and gives me a reason to inspire others. My life's journey, reflections of my past, family and my writings will change as time goes on. Being able to adapt to those changes is where I will find my purpose, the best me.

Your Journey

It is our journey, where we stumble and recover, the mistakes we make and correct, that are a factor in our success. Our ability to be at peace with ourselves and achievements also depend on our mindset, that "madness". Often people blame circumstances, those they associate with, and family for their lack of success. Success is not measured by time, age, race, culture, handicap or lack of support or aid. What matters most is the determination to pursue it. Having the courage to face your fears and commit to making the necessary changes.

Managing your madness is not a terminology that is used by all, but it is understood. Our actions and reactions depend on us making sound decisions and realizing it's a personal choice to change our behaviors.

I wish you nothing but success in all your endeavors.

SELF -TEST

1. What has held you hostage or brings on
    personal fears?

    _____

    _____

    _____

    _____

    _____

    _____

2. What have you done to manage problems
    when overwhelmed?

    _____

    _____

    _____

    _____

    _____

    _____

3. What positive thought or action is/has become a part of your daily life?

    _____

    _____

    _____

    _____

    _____

    _____

    _____

4. What can you identify/know that needs immediate attention or change?

    _____

    _____

    _____

    _____

    _____

    _____

    _____

5. Are you willing to change your mindset?

_____

_____

_____

_____

_____

_____

6. What have you been able to share with others?

_____

_____

_____

_____

_____

_____

7. What stood out the most for you in your past experiences that would prove the need for a change in one's mindset?

_____

_____

_____

_____

_____

_____

8. When reflecting what have you learned that you didn't know or understand before?

_____

_____

_____

_____

_____

_____

9. How would you add to this reading?

    _____

    _____

    _____

    _____

    _____

    _____

10. Would you recommend this book as a
    workshop or webinar for others?

    _____

    _____

    _____

    _____

    _____

    _____

NOTES

_____

_____

_____

_____

_____

_____

_____

_____

_____

_____

_____

_____

_____

NOTES

_____

_____

_____

_____

_____

_____

_____

_____

_____

_____

_____

_____

_____

About I Pen Book's Author
Nanette M. Buchanan

A Dynamic Speaker and Author

Nanette M. Buchanan is a native of Newark, New Jersey now residing in Fayetteville, North Carolina.

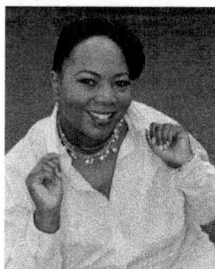

She first set her pen to pad, as written expressions of her love for poetry. To date, her pen to pad accomplishments includes three volumes of poetry, four yet to be published children's books, one published children's book, and twelve published novels. When asked what genre' best describes her novels, she teasingly answers, "Reality Fiction". Her preferred genre' is women's fiction or crime fiction, but readers will attest they all have suspense, mystery and a dramatic twist.

At the start of her employment Nanette worked as a Recreation Supervisor at the Newark Westward Boys and Girls Club where she enjoyed developing programs and working with the youth. She was also a track coach for the Newark YMCA for twenty years. It was her involvement with the youth that lea her to pursue a career in State Corrections. "Watching the youth fall prey to the community pitfalls in crime. I thought being a part of the system I could somehow steer them in another direction. I filled out the application with the intent to become a part of the juvenile system. After discovering the politics in the system, I decided to take the test for a placement in the adult facilities."

After twenty-five years and retiring as a Sergeant, Nanette has begun speaking about the realities many must face in life. As a motivational and transformational speaker, it is her goal to open a dialogue that will mend deep rooted issues for many. Her company is I Pen Visions, LLC which hosts many of her ongoing projects. As the CEO, she has launched *I Pen Magazine,* a quarterly magazine, and an I Pen Podcast called "Let's Talk About It," which streams weekly.

It is her goal to become a successful speaker and author without limits, writing and producing plays that feature her poems as well as adaptations of her novels on the "big screen". This diverse author is available for interviews, chats, signings, and speaking engagements. She welcomes all to visit her website:

ipenbooks.now.site

or contact her via email

ipendesigns@gmail.com

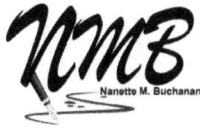

Novels by Nanette M. Buchanan

Family Secrets Lies and Alibi's

A Different Kind of Love

Bruised Love

Skeletons Beyond The Closed Door

Gossip Line

Bonded Betrayal

Scattered Pieces

The Stranger Within

The Perfect Side Piece

The Hustler's Touch

Duplicity

The Corner Pew

Purchase Your Copy Today

www.NanetteMBuchanan.com

*Books are available in Kindle, Nook
and other ebook formats*

www.ingramcontent.com/pod-product-compliance
Lightning Source LLC
Chambersburg PA
CBHW071115030426
42336CB00013BA/2094